it doesn't
count *if*...

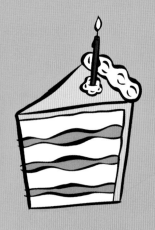

it doesn't *if...*
count

it's the last one

And 204 More Reasons Why You Can Eat That

Daisy Westmoor

ILLUSTRATIONS BY
MARY LYNN BLASUTTA

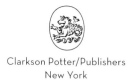

Clarkson Potter/Publishers
New York

Copyright © 2008 by Clarkson Potter/Publishers, an imprint of the
Crown Publishing Group, a division of Random House, Inc., New York

Illustrations by Mary Lynn Blasutta

Published in the United States by Clarkson Potter/Publishers,
an imprint of the Crown Publishing Group, a division of Random
House, Inc., New York.
www.crownpublishing.com
www.clarksonpotter.com

CLARKSON POTTER is a trademark and POTTER with colophon is a
registered trademark of Random House, Inc.

Library of Congress Cataloging-in-Publication Data
Westmoor, Daisy.

It doesn't count if...: it's the last one/Daisy Westmoor—1st ed.
          p. cm.

1. Reducing diets—Humor. I. Title. II. Title: It does not count if—.

PN6231.D64W44 2008
613.2'50207—dc22
                    2008021197

ISBN 978-0-307-45148-4

Printed in China

Design by Amy Sly

10   9   8   7   6   5   4   3   2   1

First Edition

To my family,
who taught me that food is love,
and who always make sure
I have plenty of both

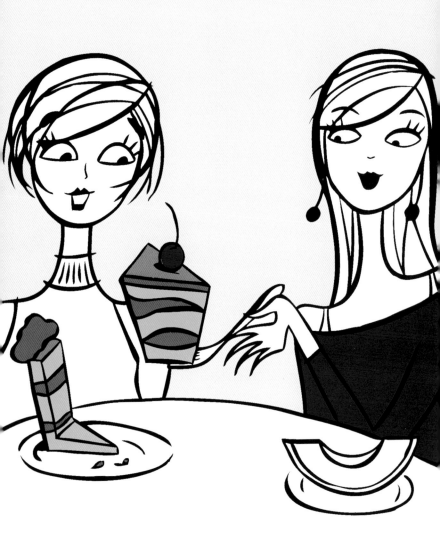

it doesn't count *if...*

you eat it off someone
else's plate

your date is
paying for it

your parents are
paying for it

it doesn't count *if...*

it's your birthday

it's on the house

the waiter recommended it

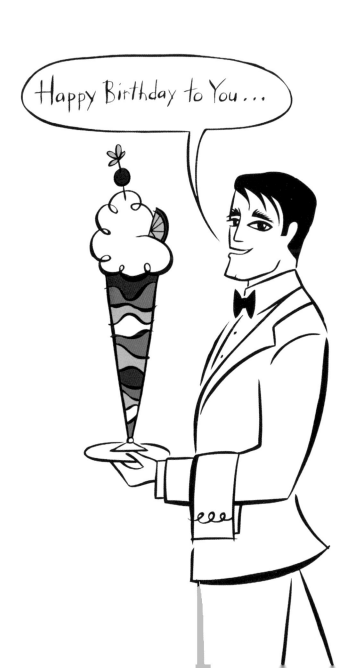

it doesn't count *if*...

you eat it

over the sink

over the stove

straight out of the
refrigerator

on the couch

it doesn't count *if*...

you baked it for your children

it's a school project

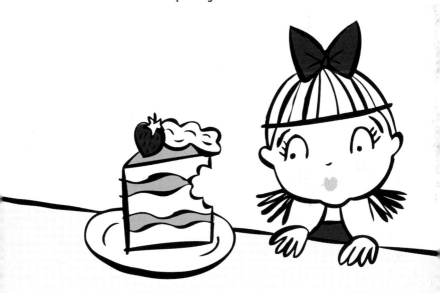

it doesn't count *if*...

it's the last one

in the bag

in the box

on the plate

anywhere else

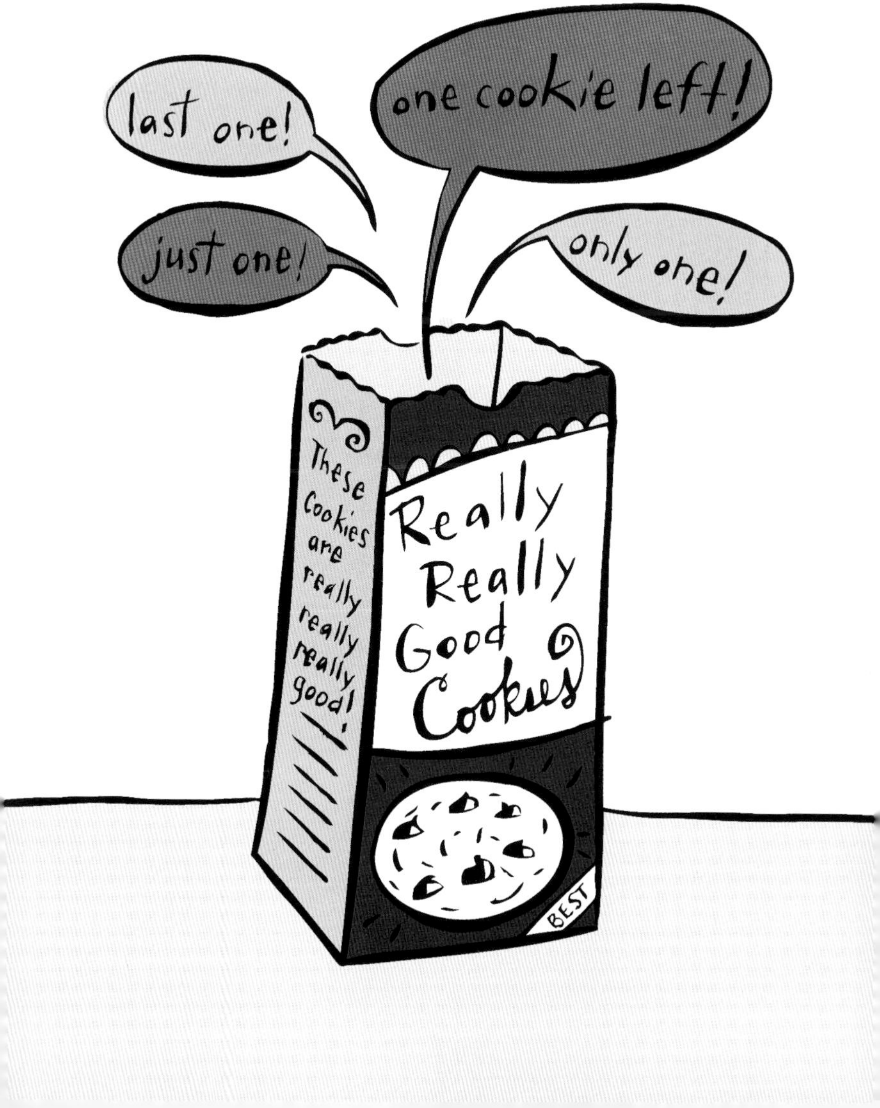
last one!
one cookie left!
just one!
only one!
These Cookies are really really really good!
Really Really Good Cookies
BEST

it doesn't count *if*...

you eat it with your fingers

you drink it straight
from the carton

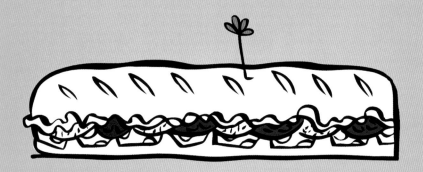

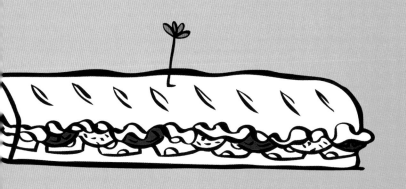

you break it in half

it doesn't count *if...*

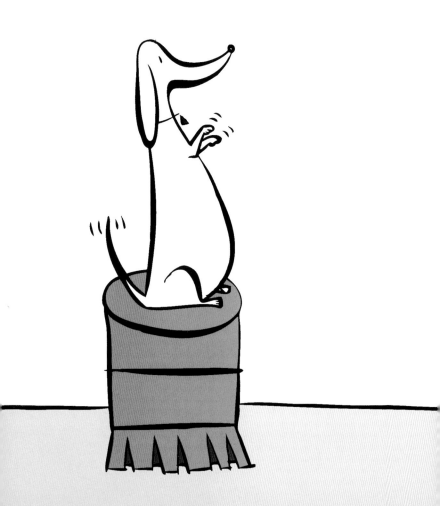

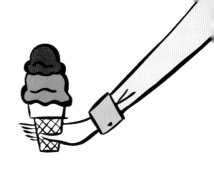

you share it with your

dog

iguana

dingo

pot-bellied pig

wild _____

it doesn't count *if*...

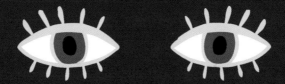

you eat it

after midnight

before dawn

in the dark

it doesn't count *if*...

you eat it with your
eyes closed

no one sees you
eat it

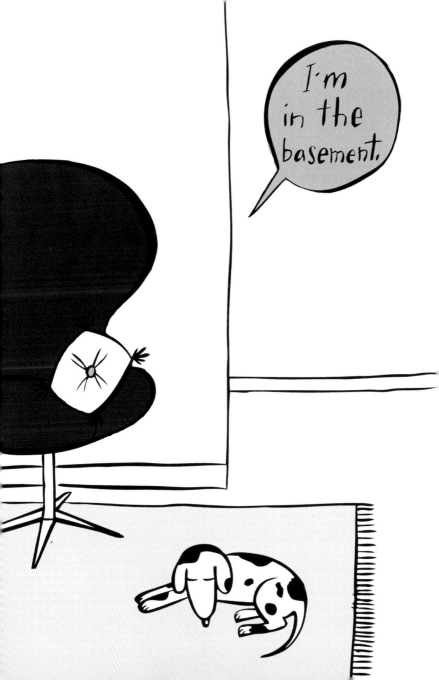

it doesn't count *if*...

you're sick

you've just gotten over
being sick

you're in the hospital

you're on your way
to the hospital

you're on your way home
from the hospital

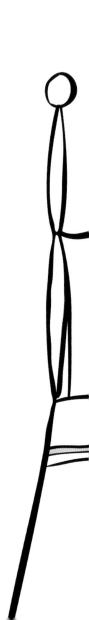

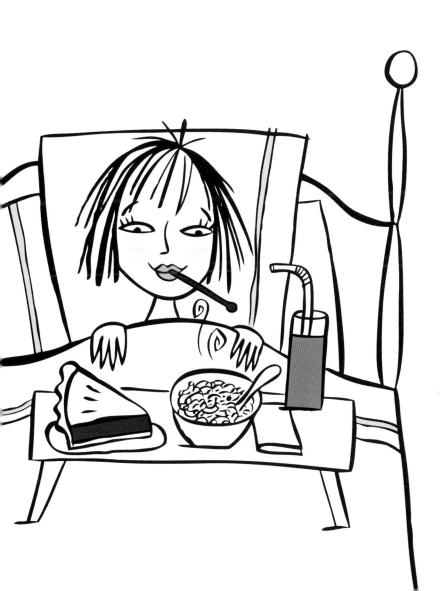

it doesn't count *if*...

it was eaten for
therapeutic purposes

like fighting anemia

or low blood sugar

you think you might have
a tapeworm

it doesn't count *if...*

you have your period

you have PMS
(or MS or post-MS)

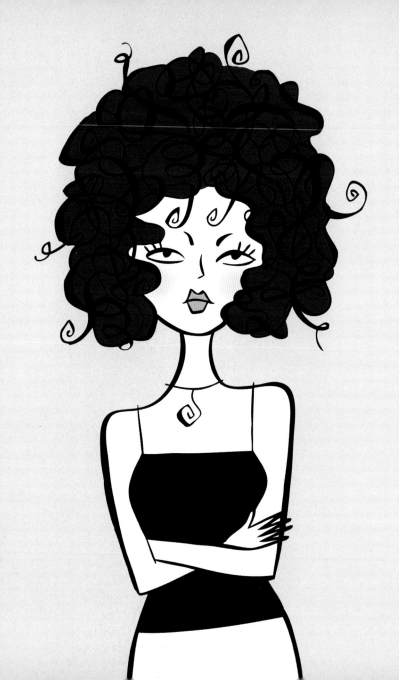

it doesn't count *if*...

you're having a
bad hair day

your hair is starting
to fall out

your hair is turning
gray

it doesn't count *if*...

your age is divisible by two,
or an odd number

it doesn't count *if...*

    you received it as a
    romantic gesture

    you received it as an apology

    you received it as a gift
    of gratitude

    you received it as a bribe

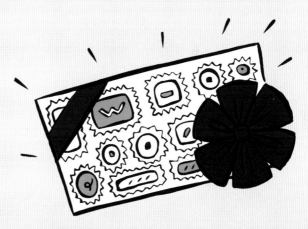

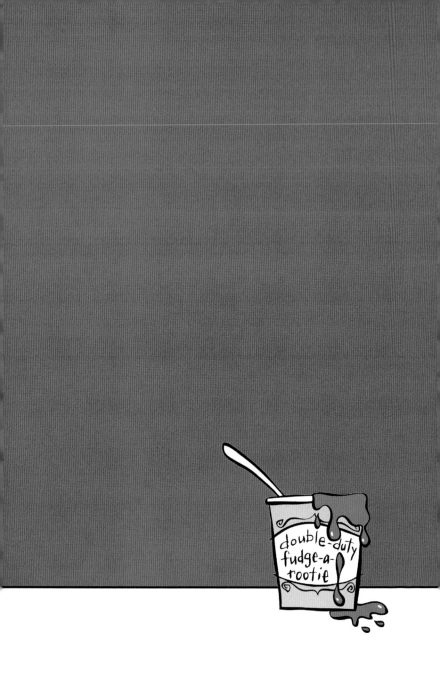

it doesn't count *if...*

you just broke up with
your boyfriend

you've just been dumped

it doesn't count *if*...

you actually consume it
at the gym

you consume it in
workout wear

you've exercised anytime
within twelve hours
of eating it

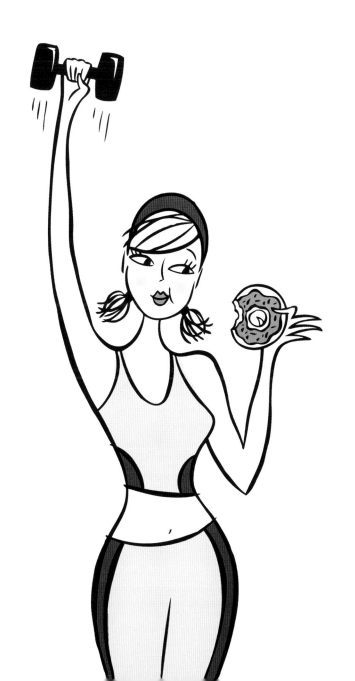

it doesn't count *if...*

you eat it while
watching other people

work out

play in the Super Bowl

run a marathon

march in a parade

or if you eat it while watching
a movie

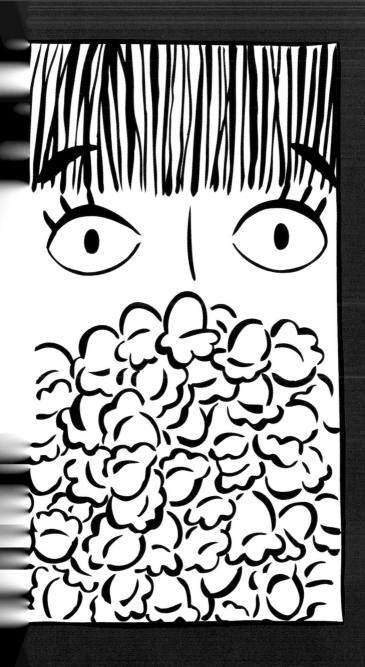

it doesn't count *if*...

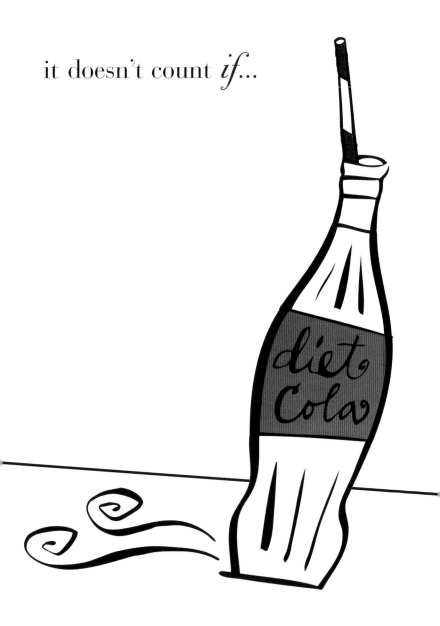

you chase it

with a diet cola

with 32 ounces of water

with tequila

with turpentine

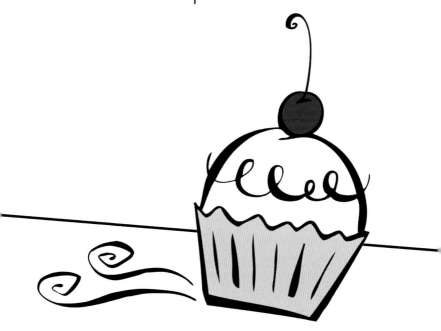

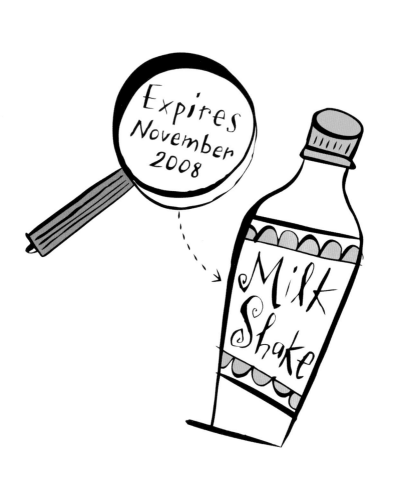

it doesn't count *if...*

it's stale

it's past its expiration date

you dropped it on the floor

it doesn't count *if*...

you found it in the trash

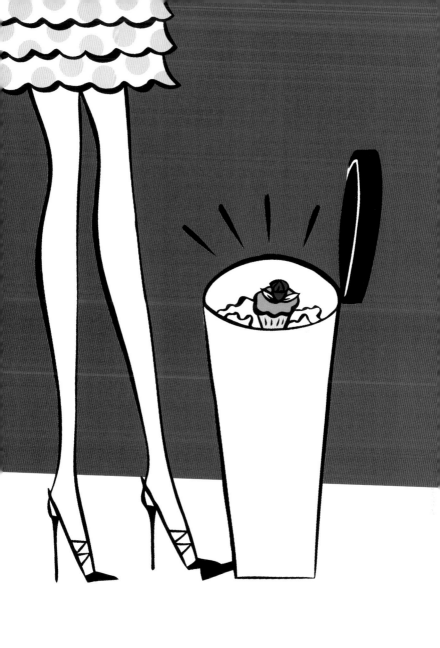

it doesn't count *if*...

it didn't taste good

you didn't actually enjoy it

you ate it too fast to taste it

it's sugar-free

it's fat-free

it's lite (of course!)

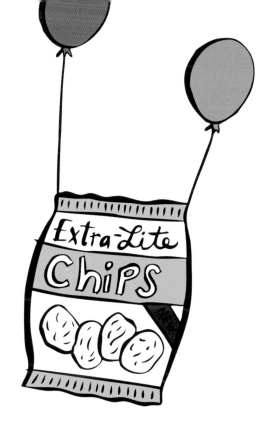

it doesn't count *if*...

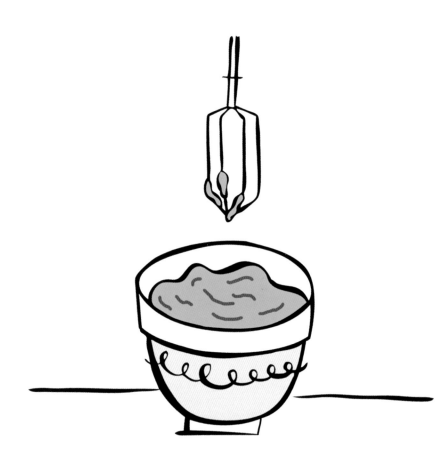

it's still batter

it doesn't count *if*...

you didn't really know what
was in it when you ate it

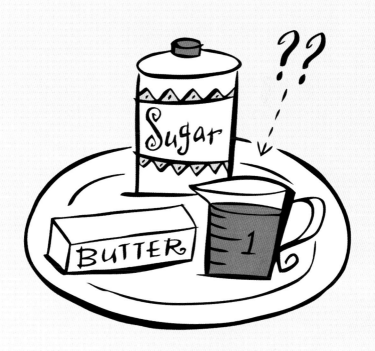

it doesn't count *if...*

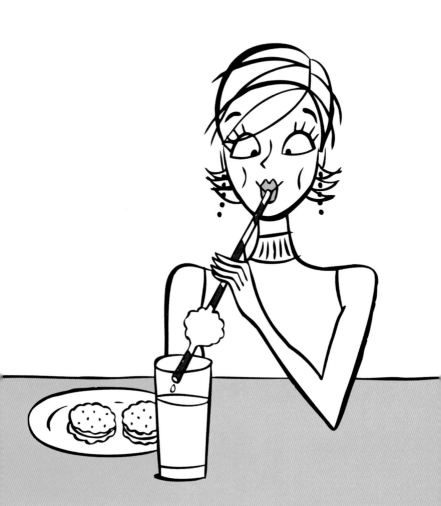

it's a liquid

it melts in your mouth

you can force it through
a straw

it doesn't count *if...*

the dessert shelf in your
stomach still has space on it

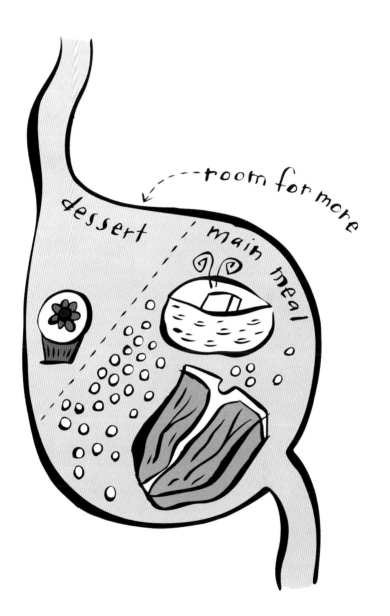

it doesn't count *if*...

you only ate it to
be polite to your

mother-in-law

elderly neighbor

colleague

best friend's
nine-year-old daughter

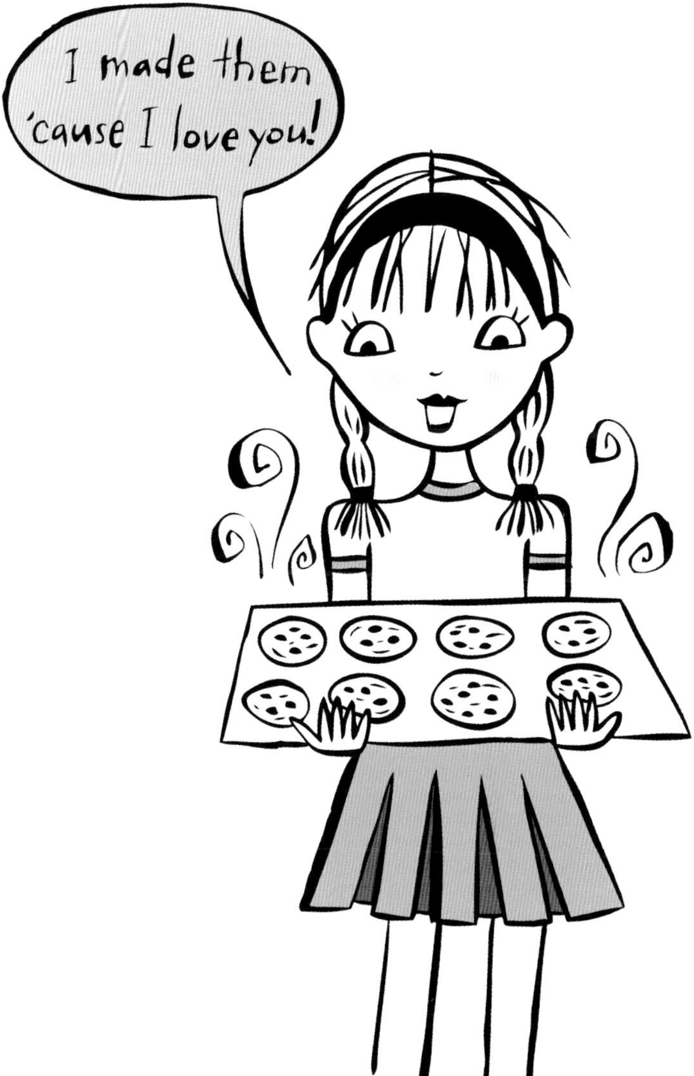
I made them 'cause I love you!

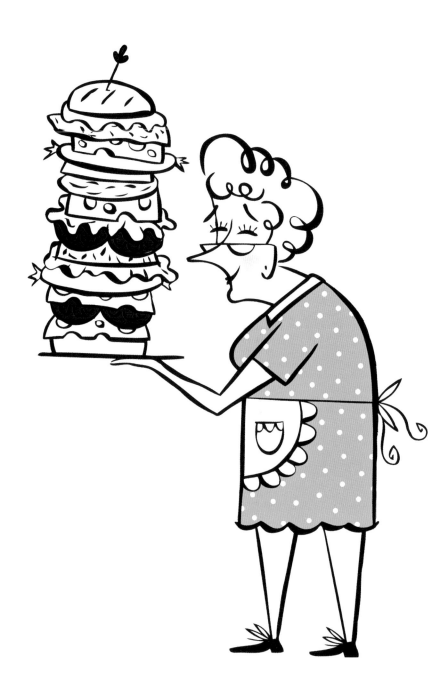

it doesn't count *if*...

your lover feeds it to you

your mother feeds it to you

your grandmother feeds it to you

your crazy great-aunt Myrtle
feeds it to you

an ex-con feeds it to you

it doesn't count *if*...

you bought it to support

a friend who needs
cheering up

a charity

a Girl Scout troop

a bake sale

someone else's
shoe habit

it doesn't count *if*...

you walk to the store to get it

you park in the farthest parking spot from the store where you buy it

you don't use valet parking

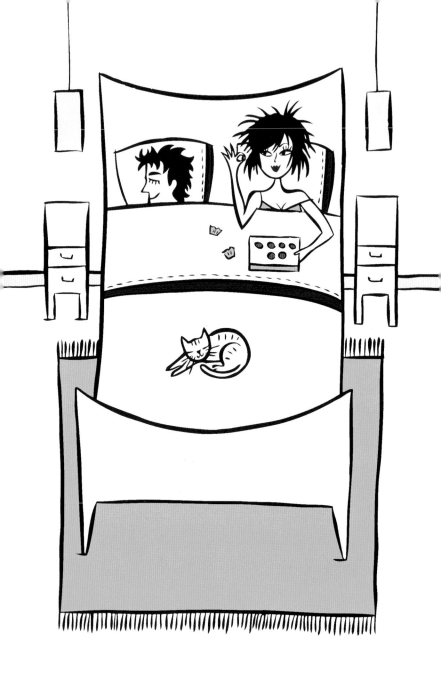

it doesn't count *if*...

you've just had good sex

or bad sex

it doesn't count *if*...

you nap afterward

you nap beforehand

you haven't slept in weeks

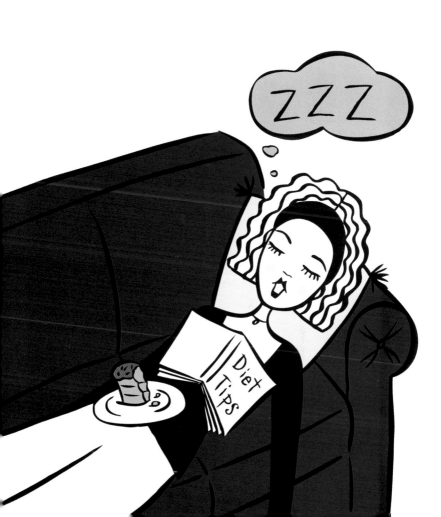

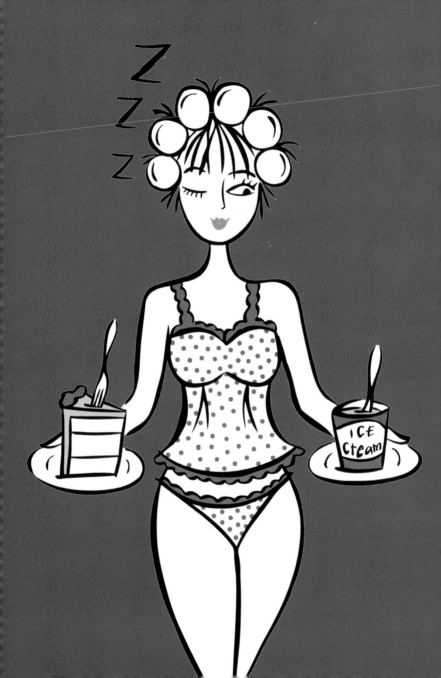

it doesn't count *if*...

you're sleepwalking

it doesn't count *if*...

you confess to having eaten it

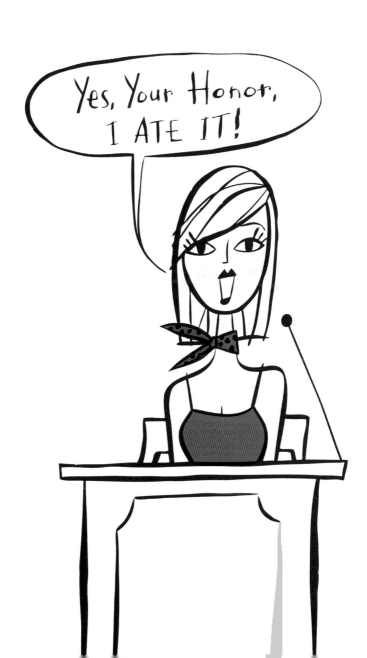

it doesn't count *if...*

you eat it at a mandatory
office meeting

you eat it at an
office party

your boss orders
you to eat it

it doesn't count *if*...

you worked hard all day

you eat it at your desk

you're studying for an exam

you're pulling an all-nighter

you're closing a deal

it doesn't count *if...*

you're in a rush

you're late to work

you're late to school

you're late to an appendectomy

it doesn't count *if*...

everyone else is eating it

you're at a picnic

you're at a funeral

you're at a wedding

you're at a baptism

you're at a bar mitzvah

it doesn't count *if*...

it's spicy

it's minty

it's green

it contains calcium

it contains vitamin _____

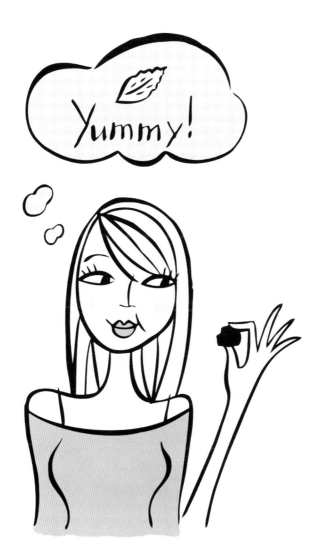

it doesn't count *if...*

it's vegan or vegetarian

it came from a vegetable

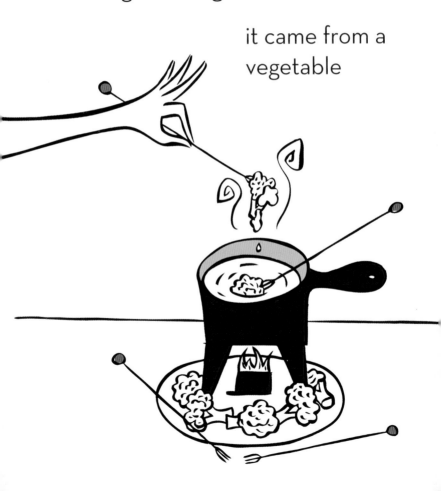

it doesn't count *if*...

the bread is whole wheat

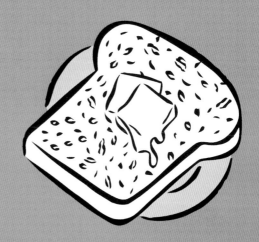

it doesn't count *if...*

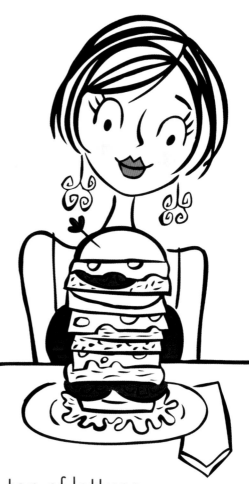

it comes on top of lettuce

it doesn't count *if*...

you have a

pseudonym

twin

clone

it doesn't count *if*...

it's a "salad" of any
description, such as

buffalo-chicken-wing salad
with blue cheese dressing

hangar-steak salad

Caesar salad

you order the dressing
on the side

it doesn't count *if...*

it's organic

one serving costs
more than $50

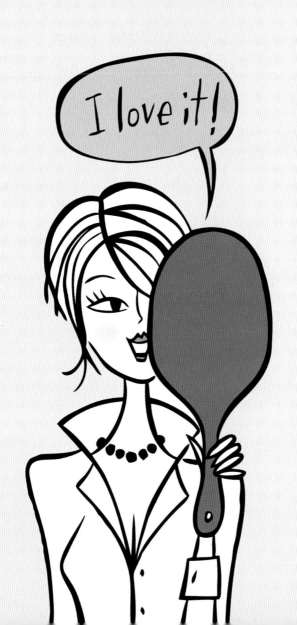

it doesn't count *if...*

you just got a new haircut

you just lost some weight

it doesn't count *if...*

most of your pants still fit

or if you just went up a
clothing size anyway

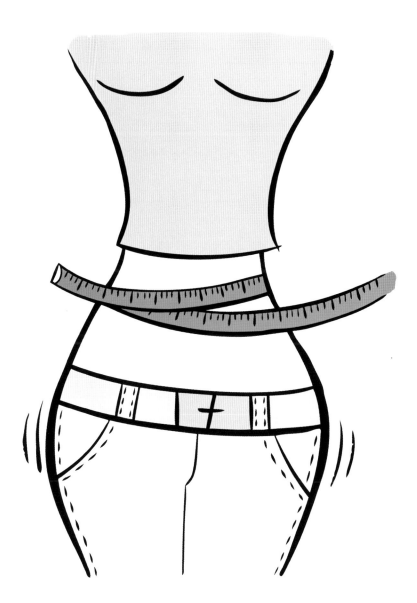

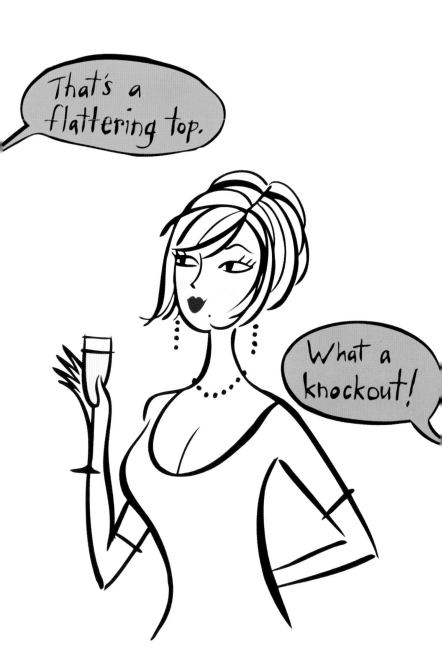

it doesn't count *if*...

someone says you look great

it doesn't count *if...*

you're still thinner
than your mom

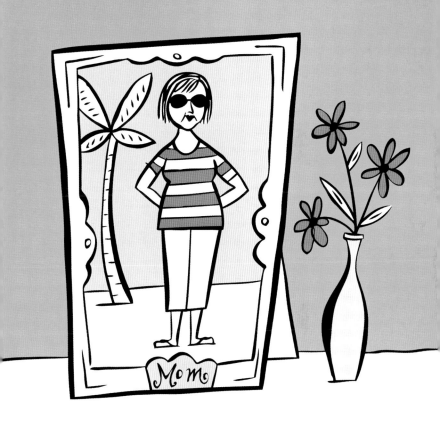

it doesn't count *if...*

you're tipsy

you're buzzed

you're drunk

you have the munchies

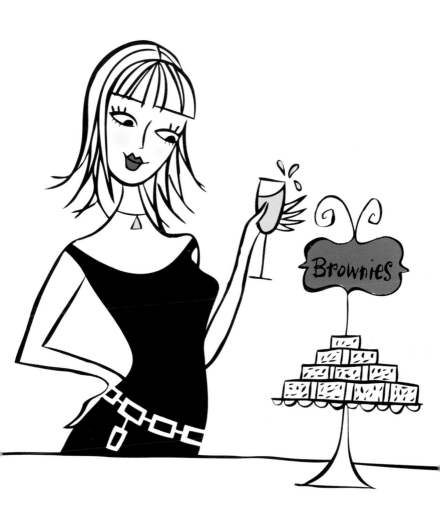

it doesn't count *if...*

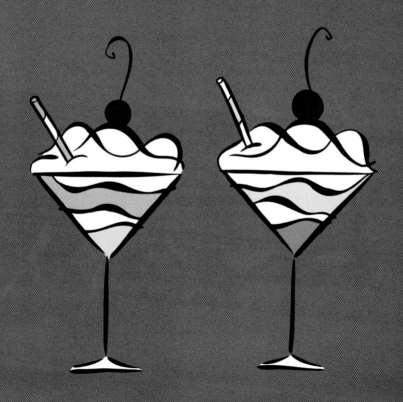

it was a 2-for-1 deal

you got it on sale

you used coupons to buy it

it doesn't count *if*...

it was free

it's called a sample

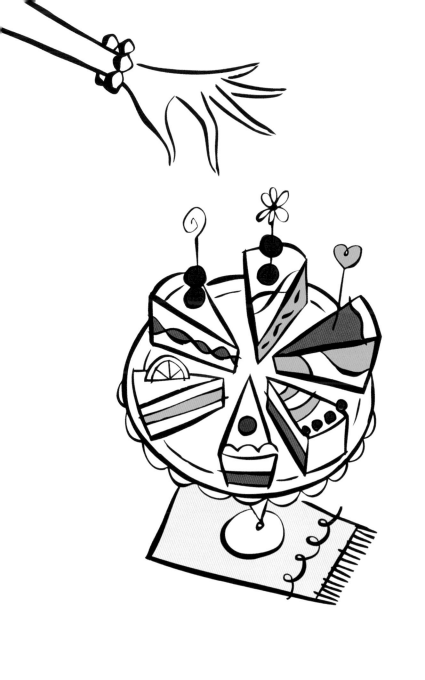

it doesn't count *if*...

any word in its name is
spelled wrong, such as

cheez

magik

krazy

if there's a thin person
on the package

or if it says "natural"
on the package

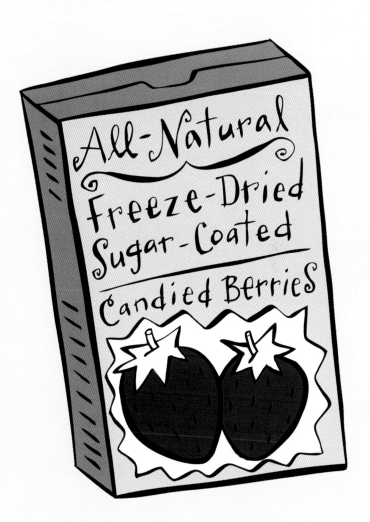

it doesn't count *if*...

you're in love

you're pregnant

you're planning to
get pregnant

you just survived 9 months
of being pregnant

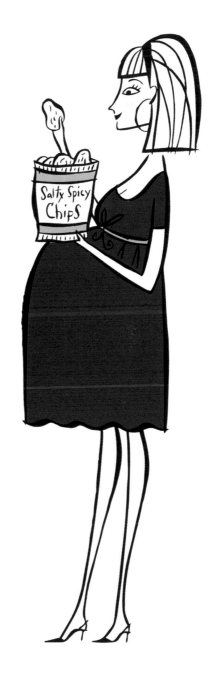

it doesn't count *if...*

it's

    Christmas

    Hanukkah

    Thanksgiving

    Halloween

    Kwanzaa

In fact, it doesn't count if it's a holiday anywhere in the world, in any culture

it doesn't count *if*...

there's a

full moon

new moon

waning moon

waxing moon

gibbous moon

it's the winter solstice

Mercury is in retrograde

it's raining and you are sad

it's sunny and you are sad

it doesn't count *if...*

you're on
an airplane

you're on
a business trip

you got it from
the hotel minibar

you're on
the road

you eat it in
the car

you got it in
the drive-thru

you dare to eat it on
public transportation

you got it from
a newsstand

you got it from
a vending machine

it doesn't count *if*...

it's below 40 degrees or
above 50 degrees outside

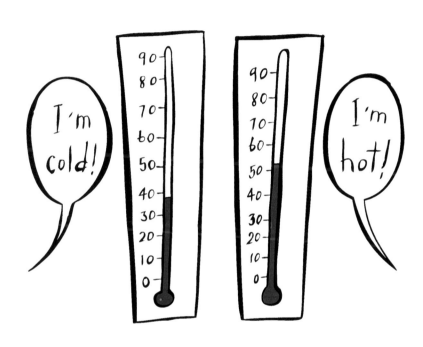

it doesn't count *if*...

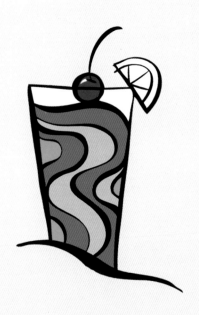

it's summertime

you're at the beach

you're at the pool

you're next to any
body of water

it doesn't count *if*...

you're on vacation

you eat it in a foreign country

you can't pronounce its name

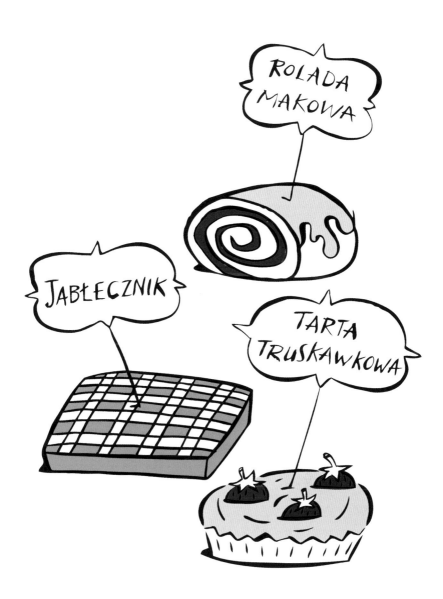

it doesn't count *if...*

the diet starts tomorrow;
it says so on the calendar

you didn't eat it yesterday

you won't eat it tomorrow

you already spoiled your
diet for the day anyway

it doesn't count *if...*

you've never heard
of calories

you can't read
nutrition labels

you can't count

you don't own a scale

you never weigh yourself
anyway

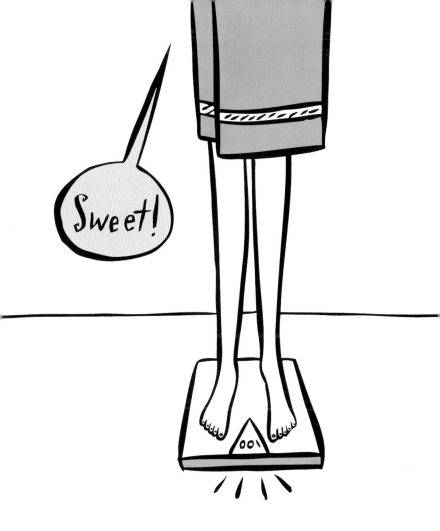

your scale is broken

it doesn't count *if*...

you don't want it to!

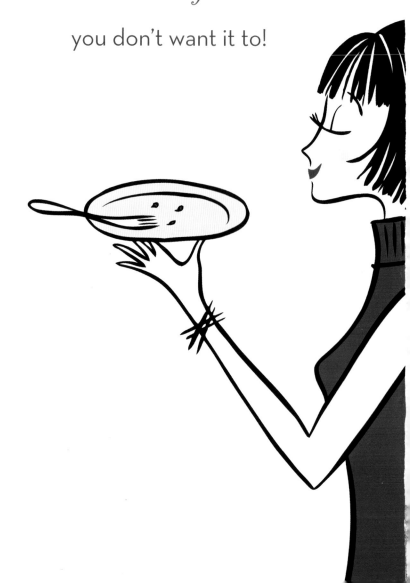